CLEFT THOUGHTS

Emotional Musings From The Facial Difference World

Joe Rutland

CLEFT THOUGHTS

Emotional Musings From
The Facial Difference World

Table of contents

Essays For The Journey

Introduction

Pouring out one's heart and soul into such a wide-ranging matter as having a facial difference is can be like walking a tightrope. Go a little bit sideways and I'm going to fall off the wire.

Yet I've fallen off a few wagons in my lifetime, so I'm not really scared here.

I hope you aren't, either.

Let me tell you something: Having a facial difference – such as a unilateral cleft lip and cleft palate, as I do – does not make me less of a human being. It has definitely helped me get in touch with my own humanity and, I believe, connected with other like-minded men and women around the world.

Now there are a number of different numerical data sets which state how many children out of "X" amount are born with a facial difference. Mind you, a facial difference can include Crouzon's Syndrome, Treacher-Collins Syndrome, and many other named medical names.

There is one thing which connects all of us together, besides the power of our hearts.

Our emotions have been taken through a lot of ups and downs. From multiple surgeries to bullying to abuse, many of us run the gamut of fear, shame, guilt, isolation, self-cutting, loneliness, dissociative disorders, and a lack of self-confidence.

Sure, a lot of that simply sounds like human being issues. Mix it, though, with a lot of different struggles and issues … and some of us find ourselves at the end of our ropes.

Figuratively and, sadly, literally it does happen.

Throughout "CleftThoughts: Emotional Musings From The Facial Difference World," I share from my own experiences. They don't necessarily speak for the entire international facial difference community because every single person's experience is a little different from someone else's.

For instance, someone's life story in the United Kingdom might be different than someone living in the United States. Same goes for someone in Ghana compared to someone in Brazil.

But our emotional states – and yeah, the pesky "feel your feelings" thought goes right here, too – are connecting strands between our hearts, spirits, and souls.

As you will see throughout "CleftThoughts," our facial differences do NOT define us at all. There are many people around the world who look to simply navigate each day as pain free as possible. We've had enough pain in our lives for one lifetime.

We, though, have one thing in common: A deep desire to love and be loved; a strength which comes either from faith in God or dogged determination; and a power to push through any obstacle and come out victorious.

To be clear, this collection of meditations and essays are meant to offer the international facial difference one way to heal from our damaged emotional states.

As I've stated in my podcast "CleftCast," the singular goal of it has been toward healing the emotional well-being of children, adults, and parents in the cleft, craniofacial, and facial difference community around the world.

"CleftThoughts" expands on that mission through this book.

What you hold in your hands is not just another book. No, I'd suggest it is a balm from my heart to yours. If you are part of the international facial difference community, then may these words provide a salve and comfort every day. These words are not always sweet; in fact, there's some tough talk in here.

Would you rather have some real talk or make-believe stuff? I thought you'd appreciate honesty and vulnerability.

I do, too…even when it is messy.

If you are a family member or friend of someone in this community, then you too will find value in "CleftThoughts." It could provide you with an expressway into our hearts, a way to make sense of things when you can't make sense of them.

So here you are…and here I am.

Read "CleftThoughts" with an open mind and may we all find a deeper well of healing, wholeness, and compassion for humanity.

Every minute counts…and you are loved.

Grace and peace,

Joe Rutland

The Big "Why"

It all started at a workshop in 2008.

Myself, along with 10-12 other people, gathered during the spring of that year in Houston. It was what I call "soul work" of the highest regard.

One of the pieces during this "soul work" was to think of something so big, so far out of my comfort zone, that it would potentially be a calling upon my life.

(At least THAT'S how I remember part of this exercise.)

We were all asked to close our eyes, take some deep breaths, and visualize what – with the help of the collective consciousness of the Universe – this might be.

Honestly, I had no clue.

But I went along with the exercise.

After a few minutes, we were asked to sit up and write down what came to our minds and hearts.

I remember reaching over for a pen and piece of paper which had been placed by my side while my eyes were closed.

As a writer, things come rather easily – sometimes – to me. In this case, what the exercise brought up within me was something I had not ever really even thought of at all.

Being born with a unilateral cleft lip and cleft palate and without a uvula was something I had just accepted, along with the reparative surgeries.

There was a lot more stuff running around inside me than this…well…THIS!

Yet I wrote down "healing the emotional well-being of people with cleft lips and cleft palates" or something along those lines.

I simply didn't know where that came from at all…yet it came from within myself.

From that point, I eventually moved back from Austin (again) to Laredo, Texas (again) and started "Heartfelt Smiles," which was a group dedicated toward fulfilling this effort.

Then came along "CleftCast," a podcast focused on the emotional parts of life for the facial difference community around the world.

Now "CleftThoughts" is here and I want this book to be an instrument for healing and wholeness.

There are so many children around the world born with facial differences…and adults who still need reparative work done.

Plus, there are so, so many people living filled with shame, fear, isolation, loneliness, and being physically, spiritually, mentally and emotionally abused for their looks.

It's ridiculous…and needs to stop.

This is why I speak out. This is why I go places emotionally that so many wonderful, great organizations simply don't go to specifically.

You may ask what this has do to with anything.

It has to do with everything in my own life.

You are along for the ride.

You can join the journey.

You can be a voice for the voiceless, too, in your own way.

Every minute counts…and you are loved.

If you don't feel that, then it's OK. I've numbed the sumbitch out so much in my life that, even at 53 years old, I still have my unconscious moments.

Yet I am alive, thankfully.

So are you.

Now you know why I do what I do.

Meditations for the Journey

The Tug Of Anxiety

This topic does relate to my own life, yet I also believe it relates to the facial difference community around the world.

I cannot remember too many moments in my own life where anxiety wasn't a part of my internal life. Sure, there have been times where peace and serenity have reigned. Yet there's always this low-level anxiety which runs through my veins like a river.

Some of it probably stems from family environment, while some comes from dealing with doctor visits, surgeries, and other associated issues.

Anxiety disorders are more recognized these days, and there are ways to cope with them. Meditation and breathing (which can be a difficult task itself for many in the community) are two ways which I have found help.

For some, medication is a path of healing. In any way, anxiety just seems to be an unrelenting source of discomfort.

How do you handle anxiety? Do you hit the gym, go for a walk or run, seek peace-filled places, avoid hanging around in groups, or seek quiet spaces in which to live?

May you and I grab hold of peaceful, kind, and loving moments when anxiety seems to steer us in the direction of chaos and disorder.

Chasing those fears away

For far too long, fear has kept people in the facial difference community and beyond buried deep in emotional hell. Fear, called "a corroding thread" in one of the most-read books in history, simply keeps you and I from living a full, rich life.

Yet, fear definitely can provide some powerful lessons. Paying attention to what makes us all afraid is, to me, a large part of self-awareness. There are too many things and people which would love–and I mean LOVE–to rob us of joy and real heart-centered love for ourselves and others.

Fear has kept me from doing things I dream of doing. Being vulnerable in the context of an intimate, romantic relationship has definitely not been one of my strong suits. Do I want to work on this part of my life? Yeah, like while

I'm still six feet above ground, OK! ☺ :-) (Yes, I'm adding a little truthful levity to the serious subject of fear.)

Our faces get a lot of attention. People point to us, whisper not-so-sweet nothings about our lips, noses or eyes, and tell their peer groups we're less than them and not equal. BS. You and I can definitely stand strong against the fears of others, look at them in the eye, and bravely move forward in our lives.

You and I are stronger than we think we are (a friend of mine uses this #strongerthanyouthink hashtag in her shares about running marathons ... and she's a wonderful woman, too). We can make fear stand on its hind legs and run away. Fear, though, will try and have the final say to our minds, hearts and souls.

Fear wants me to believe I'll always struggle financially, never fall in love again, never be "good enough" for a lot of people, and never have my own space to live in again. It's a lot of unfounded mind crap. My work is to not "buy in" totally to fear's irrational leanings.

Are there legitimate things to be afraid of? Yes. If someone is abusing you physically, mentally, spiritually or emotionally, then being afraid of them is very normal. Get help now if that's going on. If you live a sheltered life (and I know what that's like), then reach out and speak with someone you feel safe connecting with in your life.

Life itself is a great journey. Funny, I got up recently and spoke in front of 50-plus people in a public speech. I wasn't scared at all. No fear. Honest. So ... what do I have to be afraid of again?

May you and I hold each other's hands when the fear gets too hard to withstand. Together, our strength will turn fear into a little wisp of wind which blows away.

Pushing through tough times

Some days, I'd just rather stay in bed. Now if you or I are sick, then of course rest and good food might be in order. Yet I'm talking about those times when life feels like a 100-pound dumbbell on top of your heart...and that sucker ain't gonna move.

Tough times are what everyone faces in one way or another. Faces? Yes, no pun intended at all.

The facial difference community has its fair share of tough moments, from the countless health-related issues (surgeries, illnesses, etc.) to dealing with stress (whether self-caused or from family or friends). Life does have its share of ups and downs. It's how you and I respond, not react, to those tough times and it lets people know we can handle it.

Pushing through tough times might seem and sound like a silly thing. After all, we are all pushing and pushing for the good things in our lives. Hopefully, one of the goals is to finally be finished with doctors, hospitals and all of that mess at some point.

Yet what I do know about people in the facial difference community is there is an unquenchable spirit which carries us all beyond tough times. We are well equipped to move past them and into a higher level of hope and strength. You and I can, together, place our hands on that 100-pound dumbbell, lift it off of our collective hearts, and move through whatever obstacles come our way.

So don't let tough times define who you and I are. Let us learn lessons from them, and live to breathe and smile yet another day.

Humility

Um, it's tough to be humble when times get a little rough.
I've had a good dose of it today, and it's OK because I will
learn—yet again—some lesson which will help me in life.

Why am I talking about humility? Because so many of us in
the facial difference community can find ourselves seeing
humiliation turned into humility. This is NOT what humility
is about, OK! Too much crap from people gets heaped upon
us, whether it's verbal abuse or name-calling ("harelip" and
other terms) which makes my skin start itching and
scratching.

Humility is not something to be ignored. No, hardly.
Humility can provide a balance in life when grandiosity or
arrogance begins to take hold within us. I hardly can believe
that a worldwide group of people in the facial difference
community could have any trouble being humble. Then
again, you and I are human beings and can let our own
human emotions take over the logical portion of our minds.

Being humble can definitely be a learning experience. Therefore, may you and I face humbling moments with grace, understanding and compassion for ourselves. May you and I learn the value, and not the shame, in humility. Love yourselves and love life.

Sitting with uncomfortable feelings

Every person who is a part of the facial difference community around the world deals with different feelings and emotions a lot.

They are recognized, understood, and dealt with responsibly...or they get pushed down and rejected within the body. When emotions get stuffed, more than likely they will come out sideways in anger and resentment or possibly self-harm, addiction, and other detrimental actions.

Uncomfortable feelings are a part of our lives. In fact, they are a part of any person's life. Truly, dealing with them in a responsible way can prove helpful and strengthen the resolve to heal and become whole. Does it take time? Yes, especially if you have never learned how to constructively tackle feelings which are not comfortable at all. Too much fear will lead to too much analysis by paralysis, meaning a lot of overthinking takes place.

So what can you and I do about these uncomfortable feelings?

First, identify them.

Second, reach out for support if you are having trouble understanding where they come from.

Third, notice where these feelings are in your physical body (stomach, back, head, neck, legs, etc.).

Fourth, take some form of action which will release the uncomfortable essence of these feelings (exercise, meditation, breathing deeply, etc.).

May you and I take these feelings seriously and not shove them to the side. May we understand the power of emotions and how they can be identified and used for our good, not to our detriment.

Using the word 'deformed'

Before you come after me with sharp objects, let me explain. I came across someone's video in a Facebook group for a specific facial difference (which type is not important). On the descriptor of the video, it was written "how it felt dating a deformed person."

Now when I read that, it really hit me in my heart. The person was talking with an ex-girlfriend, getting her opinion about dating him.

Be that as it may, the mere fact that this man would call himself "deformed" struck a nerve in me. I honestly do not see anyone—child or adult—in the facial difference community as "deformed." If this man sees himself in that light, then so be it. I would say to this man that he's not "deformed." In fact, he wasn't so "deformed" to have a girlfriend.

Yeah, I hear some of you going "Oh Joe, get over it. It's just a word. Stop being so sensitive." I get it. OK fine, quit being so sensitive. But I am NOT deformed. This man—me—is definitely MORE than my facial difference...a unilateral cleft lip and cleft palate.

My heart is not "deformed."

My soul is not "deformed."

Same goes for you, my friends.

YOU are not "deformed." You are beautiful sentient beings of light. You carry the beating heart and pulse of life within your veins and bodies. You are survivors, warriors, goddesses, powerful beyond any restrictions anyone might place upon you.

I'm not just making crap up here. Parents and guardians, a lot of you are tougher than a $2 steak (pardon the Jim Ross reference). I mean it from my heart to yours.

May you see yourself as incredibly beautiful souls and spirits, filled with a spark of divinity which is yours and yours alone. I also realize some of you are not interested in anything spiritual or religious. So I would ask you to see yourselves through the lens of love. After all, the facial difference community around the world needs more love and less fear and hate in it.

No, you and I are not "deformed." Remember this when bullies and those who have no sense at all start kicking up dirt in your faces.

The power of emotional presence

I truly believe this is a vital subject to address. Emotional presence, to me, means being fully alive and aware of each step in your life.

Being "present" is something many in the facial difference community may have a hard time doing on a routine basis.

Many of us know the all-too-common struggles involving our health. This can range from surgical procedures to environmental and living situations which bring on too much pressure.

Probably, many of us have spent a lot of time "checked out" emotionally and reacting from a place of anxiety and fear. It's not unusual nor is it something worth feeling any shame about at all.

American businessman and entrepreneur Gary Vaynerchuk reminds people about the power of self-awareness and how it can help them in business and life.

Self-awareness is important, too.

I do believe having a powerful sense of emotional presence is a positive state to be in as much as possible. Sure, there are going to be human moments where being emotionally present will not happen.

It happens to me, for sure.

May you and I do our best to be emotionally present for ourselves, our families, and our friends each day. May we look to others with kind hearts and loving tendencies to help us when we're struggling to get through each day.

The power of transformation

There is something deep within us all that can drive us toward changing our life for the better.

I see examples daily in my own little fitness and health world of men and women changing their eating habits, picking up a dumbbell or trying a leg press for the first time...and they do it again and again.

Little changes, then more changes, happen through the practice of consistency.

In the facial difference world, you and I also have the power of transformation within us...and it goes far beyond surgical procedures. No, our transformations begin on the inside. Our strength of heart, spirit and soul make us a hearty group of beloved people.

May you and I embrace the power of transformation.

May we lift our hearts above the noise which would keep us in the status quo of life.

Courage

Poet Karle Wilson Baker, in her poem "Courage," is correctly credited with the words "Courage is fear that has said its prayers." To me, it means anyone filled with courage and willing to go through tough and difficult times has loaded up on some spiritual power for support.

Courage comes in many shapes and forms. There are many courageous men and women in the facial difference community around the world. Every single day, they face decisions and emotional struggles which can take them down some perilous paths.

Courage means looking at those difficult problems, having an inner willingness to go to war with them (metaphorically speaking), and become the winner and not the victim.

Deep down, I know I'm filled with courage. I'm also a scared little boy at times, too...even though I'm older, that anxiety-riddled 8-year-old boy just loves to get me going in emotional entanglements.

This is where my courageous, brave energy must be summoned from within so I can protect and love the scared kid in me.

It takes courage to write about this emotional stuff. It takes courage to deal with multiple surgeries. It takes courage to understand when life's "master plan" falls apart like a cheap suit. It takes courage to look at other people, who think they are "superior" because of their perfect faces and bodies, and know—deep inside—that you and I are OK.

Courage is the touchstone of adults and children not only in the facial difference community...but those on the outside looking inside. It is this bold, courageous strength we are filled with which beckons us all to be better than those who would force us into hiding or shame us.

No. We deserve to be heard, loved, accepted, supported and nurtured. Find your courage, friends, and fill yourself up with it each and every day.

Facing and moving through trauma

A friend of mine posted on her social media timeline an incredibly powerful story on women and trauma. It really did touch my heart deeply, and let me see—yet again—how traumatic issues can affect women and, as well, men too.

There's absolutely no telling how those children and adults in the facial difference community around the world go through traumatic events. You do understand that in some third-world countries, people with cleft lips, cleft palates and other facial differences are looked upon as "the devil" or some evil soul.

How messed up is that? It is horribly so.

Plus, consider those who to go through numerous surgical procedures and have plastic surgeons working on reconstructing their faces. All of the surgeries, while probably necessary, can leave indelible marks upon one's soul and cause more problems than ever before.

Trauma doesn't always come in the form of surgeries, though. It can come from people taking advantage of those individuals like us...whether it is emotional, mental or physical abuse. Seeing one as "less than" gives some really sick people an idea to take advantage of those who are not as strong, as secure, or as pretty as they are in life.

How do many of us deal with trauma? Well, it can turn into obsessive patterns, substance abuse, self-harm (cutting), and serious mental and emotional problems. To be clear, there are wonderful people who are equipped with helping many people move through traumatic moments. Sometimes, though, those moments just linger on and on inside.

If you are going through a traumatic situation in your life, then please reach out.

Don't make the excuse to "suck it up" and push through it all by yourself. You might end up finding yourself spending too much time isolated and in your own darkened rooms.

There is no need for this to happen. Reach out if you feel OK doing so. Find safe people and let them know what is going on.

May you feel love's safe, tender touch in your lives. May we look up from downcast eyes, furrowed brows, and hung heads to see a bright sunshine and light which leads to more hope.

Taking a deep breath

If you spend a lot of time (maybe too much) on Facebook and other social media platforms, then you might suffer from a severe case of overwhelm when it comes to issues near and far.

The big three subjects of life—politics, religion and sex—are predominant ones.

Trust me, I could go on an absolute mega-rant about those lecherous individuals who decided to use Facebook Live a few years ago and record their abuse of an individual with special needs.

Really? What are you doing with your life? Glad you got caught, fools.

So now, I shall stop and take a deep breath.

Yes, taking a deep breath is rather miraculous for some individuals in the facial difference community. Some of us have breathing issues because of our congenital issues with noses. Some have issues involving other areas of their bodies due to other ailments affecting lung capacity.

Taking a deep breath allows overflowing blood pressure to come down. It also makes us just simply stop the freight train of emotional distress for a couple of minutes. It can lead to a period of sanity instead of frantic moments filled with insanity.

I hope you can take a deep breath.

If you cannot for some reason, then I hope you can simply hit the "pause" button within your frantic heart and soul...and rest.

There is a great sense of peace and serenity which overcomes our bodies and minds with the influx of fresh air.

Let's grasp it together, hold our heads up high and rise above the stress and strain of everyday living.

The power of the human heart

Ah, that magnificent multi-valve muscle of the human
body...the heart. How many people say to those in the facial
difference community what big-hearted souls we are?

Maybe not very often.

I'll let you in on a secret.

You have a big heart.

Yes, you dear child of this big world.

You who cry and desire no more pain.

You who wish to never see another doctor or surgical procedure again in your life...whether it involves another reconstructive surgery or something else with your body.

Yes, you parents of said child. You also have big hearts.

They may have been strained by the pressure of doing all you can for your child.

Your heart may have been broken because a marriage or relationship ended over this child's facial difference and other issues.

Your heart may simply desire one simple moment's break from life continually beating you down.

Your heart might be at the point of simply not being able to take another sleepless night hearing your young child or teenager in pain.

We are survivors and thrivers of the highest honor.

You, young child.

You, young teenage boy and girl.

You, young adult.

You, adult.

You, older adult.

Yes...we in the worldwide facial difference community have had our fair share of heartbreak and heartache.

Well, may you rest (literally and figuratively) in the unbelievable truth that your heart is stronger than ever. It beats so beautifully...as beautiful as the smile on your face.

Give yourself the permission to listen to your heart...and sing a happy song if you can do so. Hum a few bars. Snap your fingers. Whatever works friends. You are so worth it.

Leaning into the pain

Now now, I'm not going to yell "suck it up, buttercup" at the top of my lungs here. Pain can be a great teacher...and it can be a real tough thing to endure.

Let me explain.

In the facial difference community, there are enough examples of having to deal with pain.

Pain from surgeries, pain from bullying, pain from less-than-caring families, pain from simply living one moment to the next...yeah, that soul-searing pain which seemingly never stops. For some, they might wish to be better off dead than feel pain.

BUT (big but here!) please don't go there. You and I have a deep well of resiliency within us. We have the capabilities of "leaning into the pain." I've mentioned this concept before, so why expand on it?

Because we're all going through some sort of pain...emotional, mental, physical and—dare I say—even spiritual for some?

"Leaning into the pain" calls for you and I, metaphorically speaking, to shift our body against pain's never-ending waves.

Instead of letting pain hit us over and over again like waves in the ocean, we can shift our bodies against the waves and let them pass us easily.

Will pieces of pain's waves stick to our bodies? Yep, but not as deep as just letting pain have its own way.

No, I choose to believe everyone—children, adults, parents and guardians—in the facial difference community has the ability to face pain, look it dead-on, and make a conscious decision to lean into that sucker.

If that doesn't work, then go ahead and give it a Stone Cold Stunner if it'll help knock that out.

You and I, though, don't have to sit idly by and let pain have its way. We have strong hearts and souls to withstand pain's clarion call to beat us down.

Nope. Pain, you eventually will lose.

May you and I seek the deep reservoir of peace and relief available to us...and learn to lean into the pain.

The need for rest

This is important. If you think or believe that you can go 24 hours, 7 days a week and maintain sanity without a little bit of rest, you are sadly wrong.

I have a lot of real-life experience when it comes to operating on little rest. So many children, parents and guardians in the facial difference community are pulled and stretched in so many different directions that it becomes exhausting.

Recently, a lot of focus has been placed on the topic of burnout whether in work or life. Well, work is life and vice-versa. Anyway, burnout is a symptom of not getting enough rest and having too many responsibilities.

All of those doctors' appointments, hospital visits, surgeries...plus doing your best to have a "normal" life...have mercy, it's enough to want to yell out "Hey bartender, I'll have what he's having!"

I do know how much inner power and strength lies within so many people. They love their children, or their children love them, and only want the best for everyone. They are willing to run themselves ragged...leading to the need for rest.

May I implore you to seek rest when you need it.

If you can get some help around your child's care for an hour or so, then do it...if it is possible. I know that it isn't always the case. Don't let yourself be fooled into believing that you can do it all.

Nope. Get rest.

It is for your mental, emotional and physical health. It does not matter if you are a child or adult in the facial difference community. We all need rest.

I hope you get some.

Heartbreak

Every single person feels the searing pain of heartbreak during their lives. It's just not possible (well, 99.9 percent OK) to go through life without at least one heartbreaking event.

Admittedly, people who face every day with issues revolving around their facial differences might be reminded too much about heartbreak which manifests from sadness, anger, resentment or loneliness.

Take the word apart–heartbreak–and it reflects a sentiment around a broken heart. The heart which keeps you and I alive.

The heaviness might be too much to bear, so what do you and I do? Possibly, we find ways to avoid feeling that pain at all. It also might be that we're the unfair recipients of disgust and abuse from friends, family or others.

It cuts through the aortic valve ... even our souls ... and leaves us adrift in a sea of muck.

Listen up: Heartbreak does not mean the end of our lives. Far from it. You and I can learn lessons from those heartbreaking moments. Going through them is crappy, yes. But what I do know about the facial difference community around the world is it is filled with a lot of hearty and brave people. Heartbreak will visit, but it won't totally knock us out. Sorry. We're a hearty (see!) bunch. ☺ :-)

May you and I embrace our lessons from heartbreak's powerful emotions and do our best to feel loved more and more every single day.

Staying focused

Doing one's best to stay focused on whatever is going on in your life can be quite difficult.

Some people in the facial difference community around the world are dealing with serious day-to-day issues, whether it's from staying healthy, dealing with environmental stresses, or avoiding an ongoing case of bullying and belittling.

Staying focused also involves being in touch with your own emotions.

When I'm focused on a certain task in my life, I'm also aware of those inner feelings which can become triggers.

Triggers can lead me to dissociate or disconnect with myself and other people.

I'm simply not able to cope with life in regular time. Focused, intentional actions can help me steer clear of harmful reactionary problems.

So let us–you and I–do our best to stay focused on what is good, loving, kind, tender, compassionate and beautiful. Let us stay focused on positive, affirming actions and behaviors.

Let us all stay focused on doing a little better in our lives every day. If staying focused is troublesome to you, then please reach out for help. It is there for you...and you are worth it.

Breaking down barriers

In many ways, people in the facial difference community are used to possibly putting their hands over their mouths or even faces when other people look too long, point or even stare.

It can deliver a shocking blow to one's self-esteem and breed countless moments of self-doubt.

These handy "barriers" (if you will) can protect us from scorn and shame at times, yet do they really solve deeper problems and issues?

No. The mere fact that we go about our lives, smile and look ahead no matter what is one powerful way of breaking down barriers which keep many of us questioning our life and purpose for living.

That sounds so dramatic, y'know, especially for the holiday time.

Yet there might not be a more emotionally-charged time of the year than during holidays. These shame-filled barriers don't help a damn bit. It keeps you and I from truly living free, wonderful lives.

Admittedly, the topic of barriers came up after seeing Denzel Washington's movie "Fences" on Christmas Night. It gave me a reason to look at where fences and barriers play a role in my daily life.

It might be around my facial looks; then it might be around my physical body. What I do know is this: Barriers can be healthy boundaries. Everybody ... and I mean everybody ... needs to have healthy boundaries in their lives. Barriers, though, can also keep others away, at arm's length or even separated from being close.

It takes a deft touch and some true soul searching to consider with whom or what group of people deserve to have our barriers come down for them. Too many times, you and I have been burned when lowering these barriers. It sucks.

May you and I have true discernment with whom and where we can allow our personal barriers to come down. Remember: Healthy boundaries equal healthy barriers. Focus on those and see how your life changes and shifts a little every day. May you be filled with barrier-less love always.

Settling down emotionally

Now there is a reason for the singular letter above, so let me go there. Settling down inside when emotions and nerves have been shaken to the core through a myriad of situations and environments is a really difficult thing to do.

Yeah, I get it about meditation, prayer, breathing, sweating it out and all of that good and wonderful stuff. When it comes to just settling down and not letting every...single...detail about life with a facial difference hang over you like the Sword of Damocles, man, it can get pretty difficult for children, adults and parents.

I do know that talking with like-hearted and like-minded people goes a long way toward easing inner stress and pain. It's amazing what happens within a human heart when one opens up and, yes, "spills your guts" in a safe way. This was one of my visions for an organization called Heartfelt Smiles ... to form safe places where people in the international facial difference community could gather once a week or month in cities all over the world and share their concerns safely.

Cry, vent, laugh, smile, express themselves openly...and safely.

This truly helps settle down emotionally. Go find a trusted person and share your troubles. Be mindful, though, about emotionally vomiting on people.

There are individuals more capable of handling such emotionally-charged subjects and topics than others. Ultimately, it is your individual call. My hope is you and I will do our level best to ease our emotional pains and scars in healthy, nurturing ways. There will be mistakes and miscues made. I'm human and you are, too. Let us learn together and strive toward a better life today, tonight and tomorrow.

The power of love

If you don't believe in love, then I feel sorry for you. Love is a powerful word and emotion which, for some people, brings up more pain than happiness. That sucks. I'm not necessarily talking about love in a romantic sense, but more like love along the lines of loving yourself in a healthy way.

There is great power within love. It fills hearts and minds with good-feeling thoughts. A person's pulse quickens and life tends to have a little more meaning and purpose to it. Love is real. In the facial difference community, many of us have may heard that we're not loved because of how we look. That we'll never find a partner, never get married or...worse...experience a healthy, blissful kiss.

Love overcomes those horrid words and actions. Nothing can actually stop love itself.

For love is an international language which can bring people together.

May love's power help transcend any limiting beliefs or thoughts about your worthiness. May love whisper to you that "yes, you are beautiful just as you are." Let love relax you into a contented feeling, one which will carry you a long, long way in your life.

You are loved

Sure, sometimes it is hard to even fathom those three little words. Many of us put our hands over our faces because of the looks we get. Others have grown out of this phase and simply let the world know that "I'm just fine like I am so get over it."

Yet when it comes to feeling loved, nurtured and guided all of the time, many of us find the ditch off the road and veer off life's course.

Look, we ALL go through stuff in our lives. Everyone does, especially those of us in the cleft, craniofacial and facial difference community around the world.

But you are loved. Yes, YOU are loved just like you are.

Take a couple of minutes and simply let that idea, that concept, soak into yourself. This is not woo-woo stuff, friends.

It is as real as the sunshine upon your eyes and the stars in the skies.

You are an inspiration

Inspiration…just the word itself might cause two internal reactions.

One: "Ah man, inspiration is so overrated. People talk about it all the stinking time.

"Yap, yap, yap…inspiration. Yeah, they don't know how it is to walk through life with this face and body of mine and have people stare at me, make comments, or worse…having people in my own family shun me. Inspiration my butt. Take that inspiration and shove it."

Two: "Inspiration is just what makes me feel better inside. It brings out the best in me and lets me stand up, be strong and move through life each day the best that I can do. Sure, I know I have limitations with my face and body…yet the limitations are (in some cases) what I put on myself. Not

60

always. It helps to be an inspiration to others and feel inspired as much as possible."

That's two pretty stark contrasts when it comes to inspiration. Maybe exaggerated a bit and I'm cool with that observation.

My point, though, is simply this. Just being YOU…as you are today, as you are reading this right now…are an inspiration. Even if you don't even believe in inspiration, like it's some hocus-pocus stuff…that's OK, too. Children, teenagers and young adults are always looking to peers for encouragement and inspiration. Sometimes, their craniofacial teams have therapists or social workers that can help support them through guidance, support and even a safe touch of love.

For some of us adults in the facial difference community around the world, inspiration might have been found within a church, synagogue, mosque, nature or a trusted friend. Just a person who believed in us and loved us as we were without trying to change ourselves.

Inspiration can come through the sweet sounds of music. It can come through a wonderful book. Great works of literature have given men and women the strength to move through obstacles that have grown in their lives. Inspiration can be found in spiritual texts from the Holy Scriptures, the Torah, the Koran, and the Talmud. It can be found in poetry from writers like Khalil Gibran and Rumi to modern-day authors like Paolo Coelho and others.

Let me say this, too. For many people in this community, holy books have been used in harmful ways … to produce shame, guilt, fear and as a means to physically, emotionally, mentally and spiritually abuse people.

I am definitely **NOT** encouraging that type of behavior … just to be clear. These are just examples of where some people find inspiration.

What can be the greatest source of inspiration for one member of the cleft/craniofacial community to another? YOU! Yes, you…the one that's going through the surgeries or the one that's been through the surgeries, the doctor's appointments, life's triumphs and disappointments. YOU are the next man or woman up to take the stage of life and pave the way for others that come along in your footsteps.

YOU are an inspiration.

I am an inspiration.

We are all inspirations for one another…and, from my perspective, all of us have a little bit of light within us all to share with others. How bright or how dim that light is can pretty much be up to us and how we're taking care of ourselves.

For the little kids and young children, just being themselves and allowing them to have the space to grow up as naturally as possible…that gives them safety and protection to be light.

For the young adults and teenagers trying to find their path in life, just figuring out what they want to do with their lives in this moment can be inspirational to others watching them from a distance.

For the adults in the 20-30-40 year old range, just staying healthy, getting the help you might need to figure out if this is the path of life to follow or is another one calling y0u … when people watch and observe you move through life with as much dignity and honor as possible, they are inspired.

For the older adults (OK friends, that mean's 50 and up), did you ever consider that your journey can help others in the cleft/craniofacial community grow and become the women and men to support those that are still figuring out their path? YES!

So why are candles burning at the top of this blog post, you might ask. I choose to see light as a metaphor for inspiration. Candlelight, for centuries, has been symbolic of inspiration in times of solitude. Nature is pretty damned good, too, for inspiration. Look up into the skies … see mountains … breathe in fresh air … smell the sweet, cleansing aroma of rain … these touch our senses and even go deeper.

Be the best YOU that you can be today and every day. Trust me, people … YOU are an inspiration.

Surrender your fears about your looks

Digging deep within ourselves, what is truly there but love? Actually, there is a whole lot more for those of us in the facial difference community.

Fears, anger, resentments, doubt and even a lack of faith in ourselves and others pop up and take us out of the present moment. What if you and I made a commitment to return to love on a daily basis and surrendered our fears?

One of the big ones is how we look to others or how others see us. Many children and young adults might have grown up with the other people's voices asking about their looks, what happened to them, etc. Not many heard, "Ah, what a beautiful child you have, sir or ma'am." The words, cutting and biting at the same time, leave deep emotional wounds that are carried around like a huge bag of shame.

Your looks. My looks. My nose is a little off center. My lips are a little bit off center. Forget that! I look great. You do, too. The pesky fears over my outer looks hardly compare to what my deepest insides look like…and that is (for the most part) a beautiful place.

In the facial difference community, we do have a bit of a right to be scared – at times – about what others say about our looks. Yet allowing these ill-informed people to dominate our thoughts, feelings and actions becomes totally paralyzing and is unhealthy for our souls.

May I invite you to surrender your fears about your looks? You do look fantastic. Yes, you do "look mah-velous" as comedian Billy Crystal would say in his famous Fernando Lamas impression.

Today, just for this moment in time, I hope you allow your hearts to not be filled with fear and troubles. You do look beautiful and have a beautiful face. Now go show the world that our facial differences do not define us as people. You are worth it.

Smile a little more

While it is difficult at times to smile, whether it is because of dealing with surgeries, life issues or difficult emotions, there is something warm and compassionate you do toward yourself when it comes to smiling.

It is something that I have a hard time doing in my life because I do have a tendency to take everything so seriously. A number of weeks ago, I had a chance to be around a couple that held a special balance between having fun and being responsible. They could laugh with their kids while also maintaining a sense of handling moments that would cause others to stress or freak out.

They laughed a lot, too.

In this facial difference world, there's always so damned much to be serious about. Yet I do know that parents and children alike do their best to find moments of happiness.

I'd just like to encourage all of the children, adults and parents within the cleft, craniofacial and facial difference community around the world to … hopefully … smile a little more today and every day.

Happiness is important. It's not something to throw out the door or forget about. Not in the least. You are as just as deserving of happiness as myself. We've been through our tough roads and journeys. Give yourself a break and smile, feel happy and know that you are loved.

Essays For The Journey

Hospitals need more information

I've noticed some things recently about parents going to the hospital and not getting enough information from the hospitals.

This includes information about how to take care of their children when they are born.

In one woman's case, she went to the hospital, had her child and all she received on a piece of paper–telling her that her child had a cleft palate.

That was it. They didn't give her any information about organizations or any craniofacial specialist or anything like that. As far as I know, all she got was a piece of paper that said, your child has a cleft palate…and that's it…from the hospital. That is not good. And that is not what I believe the majority of healthcare professionals at hospitals would do. I may be wrong.

So, what I want to do here is simply address the issue for healthcare providers around the world.

First off, if you're a hospital, and you have a parent that gives birth to a child with a craniofacial anomaly and you're giving them a piece of paper that says "this is what it is" and giving it to them, and that's it?

That is not good procedure; it is not good, and I'll tell you why. Because the parents may not be aware, OK, that their child has a facial difference. They may not have the ability, in some places, to get ultrasounds done so that they'd get some knowledge and awareness that their child has a facial difference.

The parent may not want to know and that's fine. It's their choice. I'm not getting into that discussion. I'm talking, though, about the hospital's responsibility. Then they feel that they've done their due diligence by saying, "Here, this is what your child has," a piece of paper and thank you.

No, the step further is to provide them with the information needed so they can go find the resources to help their child.

Plus, they can help themselves as their child goes about getting the needed care.

Don't just give them a piece of paper saying "this is what it is" and say good-bye. If you're a hospital or healthcare provider and you don't know where to get the information, then I'm going to make some suggestions here.

You can at least start here, OK, with this organization. Start here and seek support. Seek the information you need; it might be there.

Get the information that parents need for their children in their first three to six months. It's even more critical before the child is born, if it can be possible, to get them that information.

Third, this is not the way to bring a beloved being of life into the world. By just getting the parents to pay up for their hospital bill and out the door you go? No, no, no.

So, when you parents have this situation occur it is vital that you let others–beyond the hospital, organization, healthcare provider–know this is what you received. And, I'll tell you why.

That healthcare provider needs to be called out for what they did. So then they can be responsible now and in the future for getting the best information out there for parents. And, this is not...you know, and trust me, emotions coming into play and you're going to want to go full-bore and blast away at hospitals and healthcare providers.

I understand that. But you do need to call your own department of health or organization in your city, state, nation, or province.

Tell them, "This is what they gave me, and it's not enough. I want you to know this is what I got from this healthcare provider. And I want you to reach out and connect with them and see if you can help."

And if that department of health doesn't know what you're talking about, or doesn't want to budge, then you can seek other actions to take, maybe a higher governmental level.

There are resources available for you to use around the well-being of your child.

So, I'm going to offer a couple of ideas and a reference for solutions. Take what you like and leave the rest, as the old saying goes.

First, make sure that your child is taken care of. Make sure that whatever support that child needs you could get to take care of that child as soon as possible.

Second, make sure that as a parent you have a support group around you. If your family isn't supportive for some reason, then reach out for a friend or community resource.

Ask for help, OK, because, you're going to need the support from the people around you to be there to help you.

Whether you are a single parent, married couple, divorced, whatever the case may be, you're going to need support.

This is not the time for you to be "brave" and go it alone. No, it's time for Y-O-U to reach out and ask for help.

Second, stay calm and serene in moments like these. I know some of you might be saying, "Ah, I don't want to talk about it, uh, I got things to do, I don't know how to be calm and serene, and all that garbage."

If you're operating emotionally and mentally from a scattered brain, then you're not able to focus on your own well-being.

For some, this situation is going to harm your child. I know you don't want that to happen. You just want to love your child. Make sure that the child gets all the care he or she needs.

Yes, I know that your child may have other issues besides the facial difference. I'm aware of that.

It may be so. That adds more to your plate to take care of. And, being calm and serene may not matter. Yet, I want to encourage you to take time out for you.

Especially during these times when you're really in need of support and help.

Reach out to AmeriFace®. AmeriFace is 100 percent global and a volunteer-run organization by Debbie Oliver. I know Debbie personally and she works a lot in mission and service for parents and children alike. I mean she's been doing this for a while a long time.

The website is www.ameriface.org.

There are resources out there. If the hospital gives you a sheet of paper, then I'll bet you a dollar they need more information.

Breaking the shame cycle

There is a wonderful person who has done a lot of research on the topic of shame, and her name is Dr. Brené Brown.

She is a vulnerability expert at the University of Houston in Houston, Texas. This is something on Brown's work I want to share with you–this is from a great video, something she shared during a conversation with Oprah Winfrey–and it's about shame.

Brown has been researching shame and vulnerability and its impact on lives for more than a decade. These are three qualities Brown says people who have "high levels of shame resilience"–meaning they can acknowledge and move through shame–have a few things in common.

We can follow their lead by taking these three steps, according to Brown.

One, just talk to yourself like you would talk to someone you love. "I would say to myself, 'God, you're so stupid, Brené,'" Brown says, "I would never talk to my kids that way."

Two, reach out to someone you trust.

Three, tell your story.

"Shame cannot survive being spoken," Brown says.

I really encourage anyone that has an issue with shame to read her work.

Look up her website…look up her information because she really, really does great work. She has helped me a lot in my own life path of overcoming shame.

There are two things about shame that, especially for those in the facial difference community, we can look at and consider.

There is shame and guilt.

Shame is the feeling or statement of "I am bad."

Guilt is the statement or the feeling of "I did something wrong."

In my experience around shame, it is really complex.

I get very judgmental about myself. I'm a recovering perfectionist…everything just has to be "exactly" right. Even when I muck it up, I "have believed" I should beat myself over it for my mistakes whether they be huge or little.

Shame steps in the door, and says that Joe is bad. I can't get a checkbook account straight, and that's true. You know, I can't do this, do the other, I'm worthless, I'm not worthy. I'll never find a loving partner. I'm not worthy of any goodness…I'm not…and it goes on and on and on.

I just create a cluster in the head that is totally messed up, and it's this this yucky kind of intrinsic thing.

Have you ever seen the movie "Ghostbusters"? The slime monster that slams right into Bill Murray and leaves goo on his character?

It's kind of like shame, like this goo all over and I can't shake the crap off of me–like "get off me shame"–and it just clings.

I cannot get rid of it, and shame just gets more crippling.

It's a vicious cycle that just repeats itself.

The worthiness is truly mine, yours and ours in the facial difference community. Shame is an incredibly hardcore, emotional issue.

I can't get any clearer than that.

Now guilt is when I encounter someone in my daily journey of life, run into said person and get rid of them by thought, word, or deed.

Something inside me is like--I feel like I did something wrong. Now, that's not shame …that's guilt.

There is a difference.

With guilt, it is "I did something specifically wrong."

There's a way to correct the "guilt" part of it. It's good to reach out to a person, even if they may not think you did anything wrong, and say, "I just wanted to call you, or write you an email, or text you to let you know I feel like I've said something wrong to you. I wanted to apologize."

Now the person receiving this message might say, "Well there's nothing, I didn't hear anything, you know, I didn't see anything wrong, feel anything wrong about that, but I appreciate your apology."

They may say nothing at all.

But the mere fact of it being some issue around stepping out and saying "I'm sorry" takes away the power of guilt it might have had over you.

That's shame and that's guilt, and again, I encourage you to read Brown and her work. She's just really, really good.

Other books on shame include John Bradshaw's "Healing The Shame That Binds You." Google "shame" or go to

Amazon and see which books are available around either shame or guilt.

I would encourage anyone in the facial difference community to get some material and read up on it.

If you find yourself in a spot where you need some professional help or some counselling support, go and get it.

There is nothing wrong with it. It's not a weakness. It's not a sin against God to go and get some counseling and support.

If you need it, then get it.

Don't let shame take you into dark places that are not pretty, OK?

As part of the facial difference community, we got enough stuff to deal with here, folks.

We got surgeries, we got repair work, we got dentist appointments, this, that, and the other,

I'm talking about little kids to adults. Shame and guilt are things that affect all areas of the human development cycle. I know that I am a work in progress, as the saying goes.

So, I am going to offer a couple of proactive steps to break the cycle of shame for us, you and me.

This is mostly directed to adults and parents. You know, I sense that there are some parents who feel shame or guilt around your children being born with facial differences.

One, be gentle with yourself.

I know you may have heard this before. Yet it's an important point to make here in talking about shame. Be gentle with yourself.

Gentleness and compassion go a lot further inside than being harsh, cruel, and critical.

Why?

Being gentle with yourself provides a pathway to relieve the pressure of shame, bringing about the energetic presence of gentleness.

Shame cannot keep its hold on my life.

I speak from lots of experience in the shame cycle, that swirling back of shame to shame.

Didn't serve me then…doesn't serve me now.

So, be gentle with yourself.

Two, the cycle of shame is so deep and so horrific. If you can find a way out, find a way out–there is always a way. There's always a better choice than staying in shame.

How could shame really manifest? Well, if shame continues to swirl around in the emotional landscape of my physical body, I'm liable to go out and take part in my "things" that are not conducive to my life. They keep me going downward, and I have a strong desire to change course direction.

Now, how do I change the course? How I do it is through stopping, checking-in "within" my inner self, what emotions are behind the shame story going on in my head.

Is there something behind that or beneath it, usually for me? There is and it's an emotional charge that will push shame into my life in that very, very real simple and powerful way.

If I have a shame moment and I'm inside, then I step outside for a couple of minutes, go walk around and breathe. I can get to the car and drive around a little bit.

Also, I can go within and see what's gnawing at me.

Is it because of something with my partner, work, finances, my kid, spouse, neighbor, or whomever?

And identify the underlying causes which kicks in the shame. Family members or family-of-origin issues will do it for me.

Those are triggers that I can identify with and you probably can, too. Go within…take deep breathes, meditate, pray– whatever works for you.

If you do get in your car, then go ahead and scream your head off. Just get that energy out of your body. Just yell your head off, not at someone—just yell real loud.

Here's the great thing about getting into a sacred space whether it is a car or outdoors. It busts up the energy inside, the shame energy.

You're doing something about shame and not harming yourself or another person.

When you're in the act of clearing your own spiritual or physical energy, it might also look like going out for a run, getting on the road bike, or going to the gym.

It's a great thing to be able to exercise and get the energy out of your body every single day.

So, be gentle with yourself and "check-in" with yourself on a regular basis. It's just two corrective steps to break the cycle of shame within us every day.

May we all in the facial difference community be gentle with each other.

Be gentle, when possible, with those who may belittle us and fill us with shame.

I'm worthy of living a happy life and so are you. Let's make it happen.

Incremental steps, day by day, will help us lead shame to the back door.

Then we can open the front door to love and compassion.

Compassion goes a long way

I have a tendency to be awfully hard on myself. This is
something which has gone on a long, long time.

Why? Because I'm not handsome enough, not smart enough,
or not good enough. It goes on and on. It comes from not
feeling loved enough, and it does not matter whether I am a
young person or adult.

Even if a parent totally reinforces their point by saying "I
love you," then there's a part of that you really want to
believe. Then you come along later in life and maybe you
find out that what was said didn't necessarily match the
actions.

In other words, words and actions did not align with one another.

Yet you can actually position yourself to love and accept yourself more fully. It will help you find love within yourself, which manifests into compassion for others.

When you want to share that love with others, it can be done in a compassionate way. When you get out into the world and are consciously aware of your facial difference, you might encounter people for the first time in your life—in your 20s or 30s—that you've never met before.

Some people may not even notice you have a facial difference; others may notice.

It can throw off your ability to be confident within yourself. Where there's a lot of self-loathing and isolation, it is rooted either in fear and/or depression.

A lot of us are rooted into fear of the unknown, fear of not being handsome enough, not being gorgeous enough, not being "enough" – period.

For many years, I never felt good enough, handsome enough, or smart enough. I mean there are times even in my adult life that it happens, but not as much thank God.

There are times when I go, "God, Joe are you that stupid?" Now is that a nice thing for me to say to myself? Hell no, and it's not nice to say it to yourself, either.

If I'm getting into your business some, then excuse me.

Look, you and I are part of this facial difference community.

What is the greatest gift you can give to yourself …besides a million dollars?

Look beyond the surface, friend. What are those gifts you can give to yourself on an emotional level?

I'd say it's self-love which equals compassion. What keeps you and I from living joyous and happy lives? What is it?

I'll say it's not being connected with my own inner self. If I don't love myself or don't care about myself enough, then I'm not going to give off a vibe that I love others.

There are some people I'd rather not be around.

It's happened in my life and I bet it has happened in yours, too. You come to see that some people are not safe to be around, so you send them off with love.

That is a compassionate thing to do for you.

It might not affect your relationship with that person because it's not going be fixed anytime soon or fixed at all – ever again.

If you can come around to the point where you're looking at them and send them off with love and accept they came into your life for just a period of time, then that's putting on your "big boy" or "big girl" pants.

It also is being compassionate about the situation.

What if everyone in the facial difference community around the world made it a goal to be more compassionate with themselves and others?

Sure, you're going into hospitals, getting your reparative work done, speech therapy, school…the whole nine yards.

If you're not in school for some reason and you're older, then you've either got a job to do or you are searching for work.

Maybe you are addicted to alcohol, drugs, sex, spending too much money, not making enough money, or you are involved in a family system that's half-crazed.

All of your internal messages are messed up.

There's no time to be compassionate towards yourself because everybody needs something from you on an overt and covert level.

Covert means those unsaid, unspoken emotional tentacles which come out and grab your throat. Then they keep you from even feeling anything towards yourself.

There's no room to feel love and compassion toward you. Aren't you worth being compassionate to you? Yes.

The more I care about the compassion I have about myself, the better I'll be able to show up in the world.

I don't have to try and figure out who's saying what and play mind games. Mind games are the all-time, soul-sucking adventures people have with one another.

Being compassionate to you is akin to loving yourself right where you are in life.

OK, some of you might be saying, "Look dude, I'm living in a Third World country and there are people with facial differences. People do heinous things to us." Also, "Hey man, you live in America and I live in Russia or China or another country altogether. You don't understand."

It doesn't matter where we live. It matters what's going on inside of us!

External factors play a role in our internal lives. When someone in the international facial difference community is beaten, raped, abused or hurt, it affects everyone because we're all connected.

If someone is not being compassionate toward you, then you have every right to stand up for yourself. It's the hardest thing in the world to do…but it's the most freeing thing to do, too.

I wish I had done more of it in my life. Is that compassionate? It's compassionate for you! You're loving yourself enough to say, "I'm not putting up with that garbage anymore."

Being compassionate to you does not mean being subservient, OK. It doesn't mean becoming a servant. I mean servant in the sense of groveling or being a lapdog for someone else.

I'm not talking about that at all.

Be subservient to your own needs, wants and desires in your life. Be aware of them, honor them, and say "Yes, I deserve love, I deserve happiness, I deserve freedom, I deserve peace, I deserve serenity, I deserve sanity."

If you can grab those and get them inside of your mind, then you will have a better chance to live a great life. Loving yourself and being compassionate toward yourself is a step in the right direction.

You might be asking, 'Now Joe, where does this compassion come from?"

Compassion is the connection between being true to yourself and your emotional landscape inside yourself.

That means simply loving yourself. It's not in a narcissistic way or vain way. It's from a healthy point of view. It's my belief, that all of us can be very hard on ourselves.

There's an old saying about someone beating themselves up over and over again, and talking to another person about it.

The person finally hears enough, looks you in the eyes, and says, "Hey, I've got a little wisdom for you here. Get off the cross and let somebody else use the wood!" It's got a little religious connotation obviously, but I think you get the message.

Quit beating yourself up.

Quit hurting yourself.

That's not compassion, and you don't have to physically hurt yourself. I know there are many who cut themselves because it feels better.

Some don't want to live anymore because they are in pain and got to find a way to feel better. Cutting is a form of emotional release.

Don't ask me to explain it. There are people who are drinking a quart of vodka a night, or jumping from bed to bed.

There are people who have, sadly, reached the point of no return. I've seen situations like that.

Those are not loving, compassionate actions.

Do you love yourself enough to love yourself?

Do you care enough about yourself enough where you don't want to hurt yourself?

Being passionate, being tender, and being loving to yourself is the ultimate ACT of greatest power and joy that you can do every day. I can do it, too.

Whether it's from having a cleft lip, cleft palate, Crouzon's Syndrome, Treacher-Collins Syndrome…the list goes on and on.

What do we all have in common? We all have a heartbeat. We are all connected; we are not separate.

You think about THAT for a minute! We have the ability and capacity to be compassionate toward one another. Why not try it right now? Be more compassionate toward yourself.

What would it take for you to be more - kinder and loving toward yourself today? What would it take for you to drop your story? Drop the same story you've been telling yourself for 30-40 years; dropping the same story of "I'm a victim, I'm a victim, I'm a victim."

I get the victim mode, OK… I can get there. How about instead of being the victim all the time, move a little bit more towards the victor role of "I am loving, I am compassionate, I'm kind, I'm tender … I am willing to change."

Yet, it may take a lot of healthy-self-talk and some professional support to get in a place to be more compassionate. And if that's the case, super!

Whatever you need to do to get yourself in a place to be more compassionate in your life, then by golly do it.

Compassion goes a long way; it does. Trust me, it's worth it to send a little more love your own way.

It really is worth it because you're worth it. At the end of each "CleftCast," I say that "every minute counts and you are loved." Well, every minute does count because, I mean, you have to focus on the point that every minute does count.

What we deliberately and consciously choose to do in our lives can either lead us to be angry or joyful.

It's very possible for you to show compassion for yourself.

Don't forget that you are loved, too.

That's my great desire: To meet people face-to-face whom have listened to "CleftCast."

I know that the more compassion we can all show toward one another, the more it helps us start showing more compassion toward myself and how much you show yourself.

Look up the word compassion. Let it resonate inside you this week, today, or whenever you read this.

See if your life has a little bit of compassion in it. That's it and to borrow the title from an Otis Redding song, you might "Try a little tenderness" too.

Do your best to be compassionate toward yourself and just let yourself rest in the great knowledge, in the great awareness, that you really, really are loved.

It's OK to have off-days. Everyone does; I do and you do, too.

So when we're able to have more compassion for ourselves, we can let the off-days not totally grip us where life becomes not worth living.

Life truly is worth living.

Let's talk about the "H" word

The word harelip brings up a lot of different connotations within society.

I looked this word up in the famous dictionary here, Merriam-Webster Collegiate Dictionary. The 11th edition, to be precise. I open it up and look under harelip – h-a-r-e-l-i-p. It is a noun, its origin dates back to 1567. And this is what is says: "sometimes offensive cleft lip."

So, I would want to find cleft lip.

That term here, I think that we all know what cleft lip is. So, what would, and what does Merriam's Webster Dictionary say about that? Ah, cleft lip, a noun – circa 1882. "A birth defect characterized by one or more clefts in the upper lip resulting from failure of the embryonic parts of the lip to unite; called also, harelip."

OK, so it covers both bases there. In doing some research, I came across a website, actually it's a blog, a blog site and I want to give it credit: www.wearethesimmons.blogspot.com.

And, I want to read a portion of the post from the blog author. The title of the blog is "Seriously??? Harelip?!?!?"

"I don't know if you all know this, but I am a HUGE Grey's Anatomy fan. (Grey's Anatomy is a television show on ABC here in the United States, and probably seen on networks around the world - Huge – excuse my interjection here) HUGE. I may have talked about this before, but since Jack (the blog writer's son) was born, I pay more attention to medical dramas. I hear more things. I know more of what they are talking about. I know when they are doing things wrong, and when things are improbable. But I still enjoy it for its entertainment value. Well last night, one of the doctors said a very flippant remark that has me bugged to the core. And there is a video clip from Grey's Anatomy that shows actor Patrick Dempsey in his character on the show using the term harelip, and again let me be clear, it's the actor's role in the show, it is not the actor himself."

So, the blog post continues.

"Here's what bugs me. The fact that most people don't know it's offensive. The fact that McDreamy said it. People think he's cool. People want to be like him. The fact that my kid, has one. I go deeper than just his flippant remark; I pretend it's real. What if the parents of that kid were walking by as he said that?

"What if the kid was being wheeled to post op, and heard him say that? What if I was sitting in our little post op room across from the desk, and I overheard the nurses talking about the kid across the hall with a harelip. I seriously... think I would rip someone's throat out. Now, I am fully aware it is just a TV show, and maybe my feelings are raw, because we JUST had surgery ..."

This is a blog that was written in March 2009 - I interject there.

"... because we JUST had surgery, but I'm still bugged."

I put this up first on my Facebook page, and have had great conversations about it. Someone asked, "Why is it so negative?" And sadly enough, I didn't know. But I was directed to it. So, I'm going to share, that I want you to, I want to encourage you to go to this blog post.

It's very informative and a well-written blog post from my opinion. The reason I wanted to bring up the word harelip is that it is a term that is derogatory. It is a term that for parents with children with cleft lips that they will have, on occasion, people who simply are not informed, are not educated might go and say, "Oh, does your daughter, does your child have a harelip?"

If the parent is aware enough, the parent might say, "Oh, are you asking if my child has a cleft lip? Yes, my child does have a cleft lip." It might catch the person off-guard a bit. And they might say "Oh, I didn't know." They didn't know, OK. And so, this is a learning piece.

This is a way to educate others about the term – harelip. And, it also opens the door for further education – you know awareness, awareness – exactly. And, I know that there are other examples that are out there - maybe in movies, and other TV shows where they've used the word "harelip" not knowing it was a derogatory term.

So, I'm talking about it. How does it affect me? Well, I have had that experience too - when someone has used the term, not directly at me per se - as in an attack on me, my facial look, my facial anomaly; but, more on the lines of a sideways comment.

That maybe I wasn't aware enough to take it real personally – like a personal attack … because I wasn't aware.

I knew it was a derogatory term. Yet, I didn't know fully how damaging it could be. And the more I've grown and the more I'm aware of the cleft and craniofacial community, I understand more.

I am … I'm more empathetic about the term and I'll speak … you know, honestly, I am a writer. I am a writer, a content creator – you know, I know words have power … I know words have meaning … they really do.

Words do mean a lot – words have power.

Well, you are conscious in a sense that you want to protect your child, protect your pre-teen, your teen you know, from being hurt.

It's a natural and normal state of being for a parent. Yet let's be honest: There are just people out there in the world that are not fully educated as to what the damage of the term harelip might have on others when they use it.

So here's the thing: I would encourage me, you, all of us to grow and learn about how damaging the term harelip can be in people's lives.

It's a sensitive subject, sensitive topic, it's a sensitive word.

Is this word something that they don't want used around them? Or is this something that they want to respond to in a way of bringing enlightenment and education to someone who doesn't know harelip is a derogatory term?

Everybody pretty much agrees that it is. Yet, there are people that still use it. So why do they still use it? Is it out of ignorance, is it out of spite, is it out of just … laziness … I don't know.

Might be all those things, and then a little more … I don't know; you'll know, and you'll have the opportunity to educate someone … when it comes to the word harelip.

Mental Abuse in the Cleft and Craniofacial Community

Mental abuse can be a myriad of things. Uh, what mental abuse looks like to you ... you can interpret as mental abuse from your side in your point of view in life. I know mental abuse from my perspective is anyone willfully whether "consciously or unconsciously" berating me.

Uh, putting me down, making "me" feel less than ... and being feeling powerless or feeling powerless to do anything about it. My mental state gets all "whack-a-doodle." It gets off-course. Mental abuse can lead to depression, substance abuse, and mental abuse. It can just shut a person down.

We're talking not only mentally, but emotionally, physically, spiritually – these types of abuse shut a person down. You and I have enough to go through in the craniofacial community. Through surgeries, doctor's visits, speech therapy, physical therapy, and other aspects because of our issues, we all have a lot to deal with on a daily basis.

From the outsider's viewpoint, if someone out there can see that they can take advantage of where we are, then some people are going to pounce on that. I mean they're going to start out with verbal jabs – 'You're ugly,' 'You're not worthy,' and so on. Um, you might hear from someone in your family say 'I wish you'd never been born'.

Setting up a boundary and saying "I'm not listening to that crap out of you anymore" can be tough. Then it becomes heavy stuff.

It could be an environmental aspect where you either are seeing others being abused or it is happening to you.

That begins to affect the mental processes within you, within me. It becomes so overwhelming that our minds go into shutdown mode.

We got enough to deal with, over here in trying to get healthy, trying to get well.

Just live a functional life. Whatever that looks like for you; whatever that looks like for me. Functional as in get up in the morning, look outside, and see a beautiful blue sky.

Mental abuse can suck any sort of life out of you. Where everything is an effort and even thinking hurts. It feels like a weight is upon your shoulders.

I get that. I'm not a licensed counselor, professional social worker, physician, psychiatrist, or psychotherapist, OK? So take what I say as someone simply sharing experiences with you.

Mental abuse happens a lot. Whatever its "influences" are in your realm, in your environment, in your world … these affect you. Instead of spending a whole lot of time talking and defining mental abuse; I'm going to offer three or four suggestions on how to heal from mental abuse.

One: If you are going through it, then reach out to someone. If you have a friend, a teacher, possibly even someone in your house of worship and they are trustworthy in your heart. There are crisis centers, help lines, counselors… there's someone out there. If you're going through crap, then reach out to someone and make that call. If the first call doesn't work, then try again.

Even if it's so hard to pick up a phone and call because the emotions running through you are going to be so heavy, and you don't want to pick up that phone because you have a belief that no one will help you out.

Trust that part of you that wants to reach out.

Two: Set healthy boundaries. If you're a child, that's kind of hard to do because you are trusting your parents for all of your needs. I'm talking about seven, eight, nine, 10-year-olds. Some parents have their stuff together; others not so much.

They're doing the best they can in taking care of you.

If you can trust your parents enough where you're getting bullied, then share it with your mother or father. Say something like, "Mom and Dad, so-and-so is calling me ugly, saying 'I shouldn't have been born.'" Hopefully the parent will pick up on it, and go, "'Honey, they are wrong, and I want you to know that you are loved, you're accepted, you are worthy of every good thing in life, and I love you very much, just for who you are.'" My hope is that your mom and dad express that 'fully' to you in a healthy, healthy way.

Three: If you have a journal or a diary and you can write stuff out, then write it out. I'm a voracious journaling type of person. I've written and written stuff out. If you've got a diary or note book and "write out" your feelings and emotions, or write out whatever is going on in your life, then do so. There is something about putting pen to paper that is truly good.

Four: If your situation is bad enough where you can't be around that abuse anymore, and you have the ability to do so, then separate yourself from people doing that to you. Find healthier people to be around. Look for them.

They are out there – trust me. It may take a lot of years, but I'm guaranteeing to you that they're out there. Find some healthy people to be around; find positive uplifting people to be around. The more you are around these types of people, your anguish and pain will ease. Those healthy people you get around, the more you're around them, someone in that group of people may see you and identify right where you're at in the moment. Someone might say "You know friend, I know where you're at. I've been there. I want to know if you need or want some help."

Now, it may take you walking into a counselor's office for the first time ever in your life to ask for help. This is just one of those things where you ask for help. It does show up. Being around healthy, positive, caring people can help the mental abuse ease within your own brain, within your own mind. Those are my suggestions, take them or leave them.

There is a lot of research online, too, for resources. Seek them out. Go on a search engine, type in 'mental abuse resources' and check them out. Even in the pit of whatever pit you're in, please go check 'em out.

Own and Love Your Anomaly

Own and love your anomaly.

What does that mean? "I don't want it…I didn't ask for it." "Really? So why should I love it?" Those are good questions.

Many times, a lot of us are interacting with people in our walks of life that will give us a look. I've spoken about it before around people having that kind of "there's a little something off with you" look. You and I know what it is: It's our lip, our face, whatever. That can leave us feeling shame, fear, loneliness, isolated, not wanted, not loved, and not needed.

Then, if those internal messages keep piling up through society, beliefs, family messages said and unsaid, then the dam within is going to burst.

Those types will have you believing that anyone born without the "perfect face," "perfect body," "perfect nose," blah, blah, blah…then you aren't worthy of anything good.

A lot of stuff like that goes down, right? How do you and I process this junk? How do we, as children, process that? Our children just want to have fun. They just want to play and have a good time. Yet, is that possible? Yes and no. Why? Because our health either is in good shape or it's not.

When I say own and love your anomaly, I'm saying it would help us all to appreciate who we are and where we are at in our lives.

I'm not saying it's all going to be puppy dog tails and unicorns. Yet I do have a couple of thoughts to share.

One: You are wonderful just like you are today.

Two: Being a realist isn't so real. There is an old saying that "a realist is really a pessimist." Heh? Take it or leave it. So, owning your anomaly means appreciating what you have and how you look.

Like Tony Robbins says, we all want love and certainty. Who doesn't want to feel love? Who doesn't want to be loved, appreciated, nurtured, and cared for by someone special?

It's taken me a long time to reach this point and I still have days where I'm learning to love myself more.

I'm very human – I have faults, frailties and imperfections. I'm definitely no saint. Yet, I am fully able to love myself as I am with my cleft lip, cleft palate and hole in the roof of my mouth.

I know it's serious stuff, right? Sometimes, though, it's good to have a little levity. You gotta laugh some, and loving your anomaly gives you permission to laugh, love, and enjoy life.

I am making myself stronger internally so that I can look out into the world and say YES. I can face what the world brings me, and hold my head up high.

Because once this shift takes place, then people can say all types of crap to me and us People can shun us; religious groups can say, "You're not a part of us," "You're a child of the devil,"; "You're Satan's spawn,"; "You should have never been born,"; "Why were you born?"; or "You don't belong here." You know in some countries, there are people that don't simply know, understand, don't want to know, and don't care.

They only know "one" thing in a lot of cultures, not all of them. If any one of us is born like this, and we don't get the reparative work done, then they are going to take you and hide you away from the world. Families will let others see the "perfect child," not all of their children, out of fear and shame.

Remember this, though: Every child is a blessed being of light that comes into this universe. Every child is … every single one.

I don't care what your religion or spirituality or none of the above is in your life. I don't care if you're a child or adult, Democrat or Republican, or whatever either/or camp mindset is going down.

When it comes to supporting the facial difference community, I don't make choices based on political parties, religious differences, or gender differences. Whether someone is heterosexual, homosexual, bi-sexual, transgender … I don't give a damn. You know why I don't? Because they have the same emotions feelings running through them that I have … if they have a facial difference or not.

You and I can stand tall today. We can stand up and look at ourselves in the mirror. If you have the courage do so, then look into the mirror and your eyes and say "I love you."

I've talked about the power of "mirror work" before. If you really want to love your facial difference in a strong way, then do a little mirror-work every day.

You just don't wash your face, brush your teeth and run out. Nah, you take a minute after doing all of that and get tidied up in front of the mirror. You can look into it, see yourself, and say, "I love you."

In that way, you can begin to own and love your anomaly. In the same way, I can, too. Like the old song goes, "Ain't no mountain high enough, ain't no valley, low enough" that can keep us from loving ourselves.

Painful physical abuse must stop

If you think physical abuse only happens in other peoples' lives and not the facial difference community, then think again.

In some cases, there are individuals who do not have their collective wits about themselves.

They believe that in some way it's fun, jolly, and hip to take advantage of people who are living with a facial difference. And beyond that, other health related issues that might go along with their facial difference.

If you ask me if I have a specific situation I can point to about physical abuse in this community, then I don't have a name.

I know there are times, when sexual abuse occurs, where some people have been taken advantage of because of their physical state. There is nothing more demeaning and humiliating than being violated…than by having another person take your innocence away.

Physical abuse also involves throwing things at people too. I'm not talking about pillow fights, OK! I'm talking about throwing objects at people. As in, sharp objects that cut another person. I'm even talking about physical self-abuse here, too.

There are some who cut themselves. If you've never heard of the issue of cutting, then let me offer a little bit of information on it.

Cutting is a way that a person will find to use and get relief from emotional pain. They will take a razor blade and cut on the inside of their thighs.

That is a way in which they can find relief. I know that women do it. There have been many cases of women cutting themselves after having traumatic situations occur…including rape or incest. I'm sure there are cutting incidences with men, too. This provides relief to people.

That releases the emotion pain they're going through. A lot of it is usually unresolved pain, and self-abuse takes place.

Physical abuse can also involve a person pulling their hair out. It can involve abusing substances, including alcohol and drugs, to anaesthetize themselves.

If you think that it's just people on the streets who do this stuff, then please think again. It's a lot of people around the world that suffer physical abuse.

Just even talking about this is pretty heavy for me. Because I'm the type of man who does not like seeing people hurt. I don't like seeing people go through a lot of pain.

Maybe that's because of getting in touch with my own pain. But I don't want anybody else to go through pain. I admit it and that's called, in some circles, codependency if you will. I mean all of us go through painful situations through surgeries, doctor's visits, stress, fear, and all other emotional states.

Yet when it comes to physical abuse, and the forms that it takes…it goes beyond the boundary line totally altogether.

Now, what does that do? It leaves both the victim and perpetrator hurt. Perpetrator is hurt because he or she is acting out some crazy-type of pain. The victim is on the backside of the abuse; they're the one that received the beating, or the molestation, or the abuse.

They've got pain, on top of pain, on top of pain … probably if it's been repetitive physical abuse that's been going on from neighborhood kids, or even from family members … the ones … "the most vulnerable" … trust the most.

This subject is really one that is tough to talk about. It's tough to even address. It's tough to even bring up. Because a part of me feels like that "talking" about it will raise awareness about it within the facial differences community. Then a part of me says "Why talk about it? Nothing is going to stop, nothing is going to happen." Then a part of me says, "Nobody is going to believe it actually even happens in the craniofacial community around the world."

Well, if you believe it doesn't happen with people who have facial differences, let me ask you this. "What about people who don't have facial differences that this stuff happens to?"; "What … what about them?"; "What about the, you know – adults … what about the adults?"; "What about the ah, violated?".

Do you think it's just a facial difference community problem? That happens in regular life which I guess, if you want to say, that the facial difference community is just part of a regular life.

There are probably places where people are kept out of the public view. They are kept hidden because the family doesn't want to go through both the shame and pain of having that person "out" in some cultures. So, that child, or young adult becomes the victim. You think for a minute. Could this happen in a culture and society like America? Yeah, it can and probably does. To what degree, to what extent - I don't know.

I don't have a percentage to give you … you may think I'm making this stuff up, too … by the way; you can think that – they're your thoughts. But I'll lay some odds down that at least one person is part of the facial difference community; that's been physically abused. They have abused themselves over their unresolved pain.

Let me ask you something seriously. Do you want to live in a society and in a world where the least of these is taken advantage of on a regular basis? Or, do you want to live in a society that stands up and says "No more"?

I think a lot of people bravely stand up and say "no more" on a regular basis. More than we'd like to believe … or than like to believe.

Some people are in situations, in life, that they cannot defend themselves.

They cannot defend themselves against the physical abuse that they deal with or they keep it quiet. It's the fabled "don't talk, don't touch, don't feel" rules of a dysfunctional household coming into play around physical abuses and events.

People, I don't have any solutions for this one.

I wish I had a three-point solution around this one, but I don't. I'd encourage anyone who is being physically abused to reach out for help.

Now in the United States, there are crisis help lines. On the Internet, there are organizations you can find online to reach out and ask for help.

You are worth more than what you're going through right now. Emotional damage and physical abuse leaves deep-running scars.

Now, some people do not believe that traumatic events happening over an extended period of time don't have an effect on a person's life. I beg to differ.

Traumatic experiences happening over and over again like physical abuse, sexual abuse, and spiritual abuse leaves scars and damages inside a person's emotional and mental lives.

That individual is a candidate for long-term substance abuse and addiction issues. The other way out is suicide because it might be the only way that person knows how to ease their pain. If that is their choice, then that's their choice.

No human being should go through any situation at all where physical abuse takes place. I don't care if you're 3 years old, 33, 53, 73; it should not happen! In the facial difference community around the world; it should not happen, at all, period … end of story! It's one that is discussed publicly and privately, yet it's also one that can really stir up a lot of emotions that maybe you don't want to tap into.

I do want to encourage you that if you're going through an abusive situation in your life, then reach out for help. I do want to encourage you to speak up. I do want to encourage you to reach out and have the courage to do so.

Physical abuse does not happen in every single corner of the facial community.

When someone reaches out for help, let's do our best to be there to help them.

About the author

Joe Rutland is a copywriter and author. This is his fifth book. He's a contributing writer to large-scale publications like Thrive Global, Addicted2Success, The Huffington Post, The Good Men Project, and Elite Daily.

www.ingramcontent.com/pod-product-compliance
Lightning Source LLC
Chambersburg PA
CBHW070812280726
48660CB00015B/411